Eating to Feel Younger

Bradley Cooper

Eating to feel younger

Eating to feel younger

Eating to feel younger

TABLE OF CONTENTS

Eating to feel younger

Eating to feel younger

Eating to feel younger

CHAPTER 1: INTRODUCTION OFANTI-AGING FOOD

Have you ever wished for a magic potion to slow down the aging process and boost your vitality? Well, the good news is that such a potion exists in the form of anti-aging foods. These superfoods can not only help you age gracefully but also improve your overall health and well-being. By incorporating these nutrient-rich foods into your diet, you can nourish your body from the inside out, leading to a healthier and more youthful you.

Eating a diet rich in antioxidants, vitamins, and minerals is essential for slowing down the aging process. Antioxidants, such as vitamin C and E, help fight oxidative stress and inflammation in the body, which are major contributors to aging and age-related diseases. Foods like berries, dark leafy greens, and nuts are packed with these powerful antioxidants, making them excellent choices for an anti-aging diet.

Furthermore, certain foods have been shown to have anti-inflammatory properties, which can help reduce the risk of chronic diseases associated with aging, such as heart disease, diabetes, and Alzheimer's. Fatty fish, olive oil, and turmeric are examples of anti-inflammatory foods that can help keep your body healthy and youthful. By incorporating these foods into your meals, you can support your body's natural defense mechanisms and promote longevity.

In addition to slowing down the aging process, anti-aging foods can also improve your skin health, cognitive function, and energy levels. Foods rich in omega-3 fatty acids, such as salmon and walnuts, can help keep your skin hydrated and supple, reducing the appearance of wrinkles and fine lines. Meanwhile, foods like blueberries and leafy greens have been shown to boost brain function and memory, helping you stay sharp and focused as you age.

In conclusion, the key to aging gracefully and supporting good health lies in the foods you eat. By choosing nutrient-dense, anti-aging foods, you can nourish your body and support its natural mechanisms for staying youthful and vibrant. So, next time you are at the grocery store, make sure to stock up on berries, leafy greens, fatty fish, and other superfoods that will help you look and feel your best at any age. Your body will thank you for it in the long run!

CHAPTER 2: BERRIES

Are you looking to boost your health and well-being? Look no further than the colorful world of berries! Berries, such as blueberries, strawberries, and raspberries, are not only delicious but also packed with antioxidants that can help combat oxidative stress and inflammation. By incorporating these superfoods into your diet, you can reap a multitude of benefits for your overall health.

Berries are rich in antioxidants, such as vitamin C and flavonoids, that help protect your cells from damage caused by free radicals. Free radicals are unstable molecules that can lead to oxidative stress, which is linked to various chronic diseases, including heart disease, cancer, and diabetes. By consuming antioxidant-rich berries, you can neutralize these free radicals and reduce the risk of developing these conditions.

Moreover, berries have anti-inflammatory properties that can help reduce inflammation in the body. Chronic inflammation is a common underlying factor in many diseases, and by incorporating berries into your diet, you can help lower inflammation levels and support your overall health. For example, studies have shown that the anthocyanin in berries can help reduce inflammation and improve symptoms of inflammatory conditions like arthritis.

In addition to their antioxidant and anti-inflammatory properties, berries are also low in calories and high in fiber, making them an excellent choice for weight management and digestive health. The fiber in berries can help promote satiety, regulate blood sugar levels, and support a healthy gut microbiome. By including a variety of berries in your meals and snacks, you can enhance your overall nutritional intake and support your weight loss goals.

In conclusion, the benefits of antioxidant-rich berries, such as blueberries, strawberries, and raspberries, are undeniable. From fighting oxidative stress and inflammation to supporting weight management and digestive health, these superfoods offer a wide range of health benefits. By making berries a regular part of your diet, you can take a proactive approach to improving your health and well-being. So, next time you're at the grocery store, be sure to stock up on these nutritional powerhouses and enjoy the delicious taste of health!

CHAPTER 3: LEAFY GREENS

Have you ever considered the incredible benefits of incorporating leafy greens into your diet? Leafy green vegetables like spinach, kale, and Swiss chard are packed with essential nutrients that not only improve skin health but also boost energy levels. By consuming these nutrient-rich greens, you can experience a positive impact on your overall well-being.

Leafy greens are abundant in nutrients such as vitamin C, vitamin E, and beta-carotene, which are known for their skin-nourishing properties. Vitamin C, found in abundance in kale and spinach, promotes collagen production, helping to keep skin elasticity and reduce the signs of aging. Additionally, the beta-carotene in Swiss chard can protect the skin from sun damage, contributing to a healthy and radiant complexion. By regularly consuming leafy greens, you can achieve that coveted healthy glow from within.

Moreover, leafy greens are an excellent source of iron and magnesium, essential minerals that play a vital role in boosting energy levels. Iron is crucial for carrying oxygen to cells throughout the body, preventing fatigue and promoting overall vitality.

Magnesium, found in leafy greens like spinach, helps convert food into energy, supporting metabolic function and reducing feelings of tiredness. By incorporating these nutrient-dense greens into your meals, you can enjoy sustained energy throughout the day.

In conclusion, the benefits of leafy greens, such as spinach, kale, and Swiss chard, extend far beyond their culinary appeal. These nutrient-packed vegetables can work wonders for your skin health and energy levels, thanks to their rich content of vitamins, minerals, and antioxidants. By making leafy greens a staple in your diet, you can nourish your body from the inside out, promoting overall well-being and radiance. So, next time you are at the grocery store, be sure to grab a bunch of leafy greens and reap the rewards of a healthier, more vibrant you.

CHAPTER 4: FATTY FISH

In this chapter, we delve into the incredible benefits of omega-3 fatty acids found in fatty fish such as salmon, mackerel, and sardines. These essential nutrients play a crucial role in promoting brain health and reducing the risk of chronic diseases.

Omega-3 fatty acids have been shown to support cognitive function, improve memory, and enhance overall brain health. These healthy fats are also known for their anti-inflammatory properties, which can help reduce the risk of chronic diseases such as heart disease, diabetes, and arthritis.

Including fatty fish in your diet on a regular basis can provide your body with a powerful dose of omega-3 fatty acids, helping you stay sharp, focused, and healthy for years to come.

By incorporating fatty fish such as salmon, mackerel, and sardines into your meals, you are not only treating your taste buds to delicious flavors but also nourishing your body with essential nutrients that are vital for optimal health. Omega-3 fatty acids are a key part in supporting a healthy brain, reducing inflammation, and lowering the risk of chronic diseases.

Research has shown that a diet rich in omega-3 fatty acids can have numerous benefits, including improving cognitive function, reducing anxiety and depression, and even potentially lowering the risk of Alzheimer's disease. By prioritizing the consumption of fatty fish, you are taking proactive steps towards enhancing your overall well-being and longevity.

So, next time you're planning your meals, consider adding some fatty fish to the menu to reap the incredible benefits of omega-3 fatty acids and support your brain health and overall wellness.

CHAPTER 5: NUTS AND SEEDS

Are you looking for an effortless way to boost your overall wellness? Look no further than nuts and seeds. These tiny powerhouses are packed with essential nutrients like fiber, protein, and healthy fats that can make a significant difference in your health. By incorporating almonds, walnuts, and flaxseeds into your diet, you can easily support your well-being and nourish your body from the inside out.

Almonds are not only delicious but also incredibly nutritious. These crunchy nuts are an excellent source of fiber, which can aid in digestion and help you feel full longer. Additionally, almonds are high in protein, making them a great snack choice for those looking to increase their protein intake. By including almonds in your diet, you can easily support your overall health and well-being.

Walnuts are another nut that packs a powerful nutritional punch. Rich in omega-3 fatty acids, walnuts are known for their heart-healthy benefits. These healthy fats can help lower cholesterol levels and reduce inflammation in the body. Including walnuts in your diet can be a simple yet effective way to support your heart health and overall wellness.

Flaxseeds may be small, but they are mighty when it comes to nutrition. These tiny seeds are an excellent source of fiber, which can help regulate blood sugar levels and promote healthy digestion. Flaxseeds are also rich in omega-3 fatty acids, making them a terrific addition to any diet looking to support brain health and reduce inflammation. By incorporating flaxseeds into your meals or snacks, you can easily boost your intake of essential nutrients and support your overall well-being.

In conclusion, nuts and seeds like almonds, walnuts, and flaxseeds are nutritional powerhouses that can provide essential nutrients like fiber, protein, and healthy fats to support overall wellness. By including these nutrient-dense foods in your diet, you can easily nourish your body and promote a healthier lifestyle. So, next time you are looking for a quick and effortless way to boost your health, reach for a handful of almonds, walnuts, or flaxseeds and enjoy the many benefits they have to offer.

CHAPTER 6: AVOCADOS

Have you ever considered adding a superfood to your diet that not only tastes great but also offers numerous health benefits? Avocado, often referred to as nature's butter, is a versatile fruit that can elevate your meals while providing essential nutrients for your body. This essay will delve into the unique benefits of avocado, highlighting its high nutrient content, heart-healthy fats, and potential anti-aging properties.

Avocado is packed with essential nutrients that are vital for overall health. It is a rich source of vitamins C, E, K, and B-6, as well as folate and potassium. These nutrients play a crucial role in keeping a healthy immune system, promoting proper blood clotting, and supporting heart health. By incorporating avocados into your diet, you can easily boost your nutrient intake and enhance your well-being.

Furthermore, avocados are known for their high content of heart-healthy fats, particularly monounsaturated fats. These fats help lower bad cholesterol levels, reducing the risk of heart disease and stroke. In addition, avocados are a great source of fiber, which aids in digestion and promotes feelings of fullness, making them an excellent choice for those looking to maintain a healthy weight and improve their cardiovascular health.

In addition to being nutrient-dense and heart-healthy, avocados also have potential anti-aging properties. The combination of vitamins, antioxidants, and healthy fats found in avocados can help protect the skin from damage caused by free radicals, UV rays, and environmental pollutants. This can result in improved skin elasticity, reduced inflammation, and a more youthful appearance. By incorporating avocados into your skincare routine or consuming them regularly, you can support healthy aging from the inside out.

In conclusion, avocados are a powerhouse of nutrients, heart-healthy fats, and potential anti-aging properties that can benefit your overall health and well-being. By making avocado a staple in your diet, you can enjoy a delicious and nutritious fruit that offers a multitude of health advantages. So why not indulge in this creamy, green goodness and reap the unique benefits that avocado has to offer?

CHAPTER 7: TURMERIC

Are you looking for a natural way to boost your health and well-being? Look no further than the golden spice in your kitchen - turmeric! Known for its powerful anti-inflammatory and antioxidant properties, turmeric has been used for centuries in traditional medicine to promote overall health and wellness.

Turmeric is a powerhouse when it comes to fighting inflammation in the body. Cur-cumin, the active compound in turmeric, has been shown to inhibit inflammatory pathways, reducing swelling and pain. Whether you have joint discomfort, digestive issues, or other inflammatory conditions, turmeric can be a natural and effective way to alleviate symptoms and improve your quality of life.

Not only does turmeric help combat inflammation, but it is also packed with antioxidants that protect your cells from damage caused by free radicals. By neutralizing these harmful molecules, turmeric can help prevent chronic diseases, slow down the aging process, and boost your immune system. Adding turmeric to your daily routine can be a simple yet impactful way to support your overall health and well-being.

Incorporating turmeric into your diet is easy and

delicious. You can sprinkle it on roasted vegetables, add it to soups and stews, or brew a soothing cup of golden turmeric tea. With its warm and earthy flavor, turmeric can enhance a wide variety of dishes while providing a powerful health boost.

In conclusion, turmeric is not just a spice - it's a natural remedy with incredible potential health benefits. By harnessing its anti-inflammatory and antioxidant properties, you can support your body from the inside out. So, why not add a dash of turmeric to your next meal and experience the golden goodness for yourself? Your body will thank you   for   it.

CHAPTER 8: GREEN TEA

Green tea is not just a delicious beverage; it is also packed with numerous health benefits that can positively impact your life. In this essay, we will explore how green tea can aid in weight management, enhance brain function, and reduce the risk of chronic diseases due to its high content of antioxidants and polyphenols.

Green tea is a fantastic aid for weight management. The catechins in green tea have been shown to boost metabolism, helping the body burn fat more efficiently. By incorporating green tea into your daily routine, you can support your weight loss goals and maintain a healthy body weight. Additionally, green tea is a low-calorie drink that can help satisfy cravings and prevent overeating, making it a valuable asset for those looking to shed extra pounds.

Furthermore, green tea is known to improve brain function. The caffeine in green tea can enhance alertness and concentration, leading to improved cognitive performance. Moreover, green tea contains L-theanine, an amino acid that works synergistically with caffeine to promote a state of calm focus. By drinking green tea, you can experience a boost in brain function, helping you stay sharp and focused throughout the day.

In addition to weight management and brain function, green tea can also help reduce the risk of chronic diseases. Green tea is rich in antioxidants and polyphenols, which have been shown to combat oxidative stress and inflammation in the body. By reducing these harmful processes, green tea can protect against various chronic conditions, such as heart disease, diabetes, and certain types of cancer. Incorporating green tea into your daily routine can be a simple yet effective way to safeguard your long-term health.

In conclusion, green tea is a versatile beverage with a wide range of health benefits. From aiding in weight management to enhancing brain function and reducing the risk of chronic diseases, green tea is a powerhouse of nutrients that can positively impact your overall well-being. By making green tea a regular part of your routine, you can enjoy these benefits and take proactive steps towards a healthier lifestyle. So why not brew yourself a cup of green tea today and start reaping the rewards of this remarkable drink?

CHAPTER 9: DARK CHOCOLATE

Have you ever thought that indulging in a piece of dark chocolate could be good for your health? Dark chocolate is not only a delicious treat but also has numerous potential health benefits. From improving heart health to boosting mood and protecting the skin from sun damage, dark chocolate is more than just a sweet delight.

Dark chocolate is known to be beneficial for heart health. Studies have shown that consuming dark chocolate in moderation can help lower the risk of heart disease. The flavonoids found in dark chocolate have been linked to reducing inflammation and improving blood flow, which can ultimately lead to a healthier heart. For example, a study published in the journal Heart found that eating a small amount of dark chocolate on a regular basis was associated with a lower risk of developing heart disease.

In addition to its heart-healthy properties, dark chocolate can also help boost mood. Dark chocolate contains compounds that can stimulate the production of endorphins in the brain, which are known as "feel-good" hormones. This can help improve mood and reduce feelings of stress and anxiety. So, the next time you're feeling down, reaching for a piece of dark chocolate might just be the pick-me-up you need.

Furthermore, dark chocolate has been found to have protective effects on the skin against sun damage. The flavonoids in dark chocolate can help increase blood flow to the skin, improve skin density, and protect against UV damage. Research has shown that consuming dark chocolate with a high percentage of cocoa can help protect the skin from harmful UV rays and improve overall skin health. So, while you should still wear sunscreen, adding some dark chocolate to your diet might provide an extra layer of protection for your skin.

In conclusion, dark chocolate is not only a delicious treat but also a potential superfood with various health benefits. From improving heart health to boosting mood and protecting the skin from sun damage, the benefits of dark chocolate are too good to ignore. So, next time you're craving something sweet, reach for a piece of dark chocolate and enjoy not only its rich flavor but also its potential health benefit.

CHAPTER 10: IN CONCLUSION

Are you looking for a way to feel younger and healthier without resorting to expensive creams or treatments? Look no further than the food on your plate! By incorporating anti-aging foods into your daily diet, you can nourish your body from the inside out, promoting longevity and vitality. In this book, we will explore the benefits of anti-aging foods and provide practical tips on how to include them in your meals to help you look and feel your best.

Anti-aging foods are rich in antioxidants, vitamins, and minerals that can help slow down the aging process and protect your cells from damage. For example, berries such as blueberries, strawberries, and raspberries are packed with antioxidants that combat free radicals and reduce inflammation in the body. By including a serving of berries in your breakfast or as a snack, you can support your skin health and overall well-being.

Furthermore, fatty fishlike salmon, mackerel, and sardines are excellent sources of omega-3 fatty acids, which are essential for maintaining youthful skin and brain function. Omega-3s help hydrate the skin from within, reducing the appearance of wrinkles and fine lines. Try incorporating fatty fish into your meals at least twice a week to reap the anti-aging benefits and support your body's natural regeneration processes.

In addition to berries and fatty fish, leafy greens such as spinach, kale, and Swiss chard are powerhouse anti-aging foods that are rich in vitamins A, C, and K. These nutrients help promote collagen production, improve skin elasticity, and protect against sun damage. Consider adding a variety of leafy greens to your salads, smoothies, or stir-fries to boost your skin's radiance and overall health.

In conclusion, by incorporating anti-aging foods like berries, fatty fish, and leafy greens into your daily diet, you can support your body's natural anti-aging processes and feel younger and healthier from the inside out. Remember, beauty starts from within, so nourish your body with nutrient-dense foods that will help you age gracefully. Make small changes to your meals each day to include these anti-aging superfoods, and you'll be on your way to a more vibrant and youthful you. So, why wait? Start making these simple yet powerful changes today for a healthier and more youthful tomorrow.

Eating to feel younger

www.ingramcontent.com/pod-product-compliance
Lightning Source LLC
Chambersburg PA
CBHW080052270726
48653CB00045B/3928